I0074955

All About
PAIN AND THE
OLDER PERSON

By Laura Flynn R.N., B.N., M.B.A., in consultation with her nurse educator associates and physicians who assisted in contributing and editing.

Our thanks also to the American Pain Foundation., Alzheimers' Association, Chronic Pain Association, the best practice guidelines from the Registered Nurses Association of Canada and the many nurses and physicians who completed the survey on this publication.

ISBN No: 978 1 896616 68 1

The publisher, Mediscript Communications Inc., acknowledges the financial support of the Government of Canada through the Canadian Book Fund for our publishing activities.

www.mediscript.net

Printed in Canada

Book and Front Cover design by:
Brian Adamson, www.AdamsonGraphics.net

POP1002010

ALL ABOUT BOOKS
Trusted • Reliable • Certified

- 40+ titles available
- Comply with accreditation and regulatory bodies
- Suitable for caregivers, boomers with elderly parents, health workers, auxiliary health staff & patients
- Self study style with "test yourself" section
- Health On the Net (HON) certified

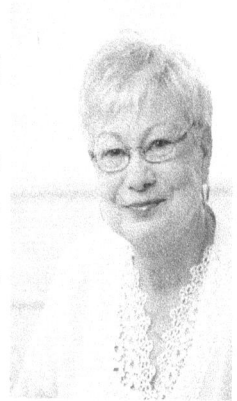

Some of our titles:

Alzheimers Disease	Arthritis	Multiple Sclerosis
Pain	Strokes	Elder Abuse
Falls Prevention	Incontinence	Nutrition & Aging
Personal Care	Positioning	Confusion
Transferring people	Care of the Back	Skin Care

For complete list of titles go to www.mediscript.net

Contact: 1 800 773 5088
Fax 1800 639 3186 • Email; mediscript30@yahoo.ca

CONTENTS

INTRODUCTION

This book provides basic, non controversial and trusted information that can help a wide spectrum of readers.

The primary objective of the information is to help a person provide effective quality care to a loved one or someone in his or her care.

Pain is a subjective area of diagnosis, personal to the person being cared for. This book can help provide comprehensive understanding and the confidence and ability to ask the right questions and provide the optimum care.

All the information is reliable and was written by a group of eminent nurse educators who ensured all the information complies with best practice guidelines and satisfies the various accreditation and regulatory bodies. Because there is so much unreliable information on the internet, you can be assured the "All About" publications are HON (Health On the Net) certified.

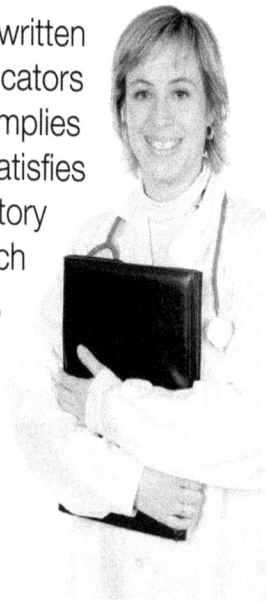

Consequently, this book can be an invaluable aid to:

- A caregiver caring for a relative or friend;
- A health worker seeking a reference aid;
- A patient or person suffering from pain;
- Any person involved in health care wishing to expand his or her knowledge.

SOMETHING TO THINK ABOUT...

A journey of a thousand miles must begin with a single step.

Chinese proverb

AN IMPORTANT MESSAGE
FROM THE PUBLISHER

Each person's treatment, advice, medical aids, physical therapy and other approaches to health care are unique and highly dependant upon the diagnosis and overall assessment by the medical team.

We emphasize therefore that the information within this book is not a substitute for the advice and treatment from a health care professional.

This book provides generic information concerning pain and common sense well established care practices for caring for elderly people in pain.

With all this in mind, the publishers and authors disclaim any responsibility for any adverse effects resulting directly or indirectly from the suggestions contained within this book or from any misunderstanding of the content on the part of the reader.

HAVE YOU HEARD

The following were newspaper headlines from across the country:

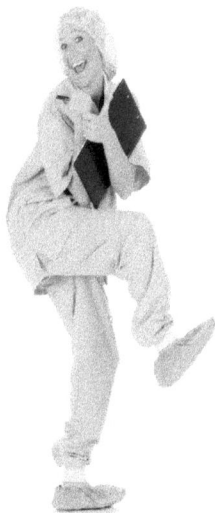

- March Planed for Next August

- Blind Bishop Appointed to See

- Patient at Death's Door: Doctors Pull Him Through

- Cold Wave Linked to Temperatures

- Stadium Air Conditioning Fails: Fans Protest

HOW MUCH DO YOU KNOW?

It helps to figure out how much you know before you start. In this way you will have an idea as to the gaps in your knowledge prior to reading the content. Please circle to indicate the best answer. Remember, at this stage, you are not expected to know all the answers:

1. How many North Americans suffer pain each day?

a. One in two

b. One in three

c. One in five

d. One in ten

2. Your family member has medication for pain but is having trouble getting to sleep. How can you help?

a. There is nothing you can do.

b. Sit and chat with him for awhile.

c. Advise him to get up and walk around for an hour or so.

d. Inform him that he has to try and go to sleep as sleep is very important for persons in pain.

3. What is "guided imagery"?

a. An ancient healing technique that started in Asia

b. A training technique that lets a person gain control over some body functions

c. A technique in which the person focuses their thoughts on a word or phrase blocking out all other thoughts

d. A technique involving intense focus on a pleasant image so that the person slowly becomes less aware of pain

4. Distraction as a pain management technique works best with which type of pain?

a. Acute

b. Chronic

c. Mild or moderate pain

d. Severe pain

5. What percentage of older adults living in the community have pain on a regular basis?

5-10%

25-50%

75%

90%

6. Which statement about pain management is true?

a. The person suffering pain is the expert in his or her own pain.

b. The main goal of pain management is to lessen pain.

c. A cup of coffee or tea in the evening promotes sleep.

d. People in pain need to go to bed at the same time each night.

7. Your loved one complains of pain in his left lower leg. He had a below-the-knee amputation two years ago. This type of pain is:

a. Chronic pain

b. Radiating pain

c. Phantom pain

ANSWERS

1. c. One in five Americans is affected by pain each day.

2. b. Sitting and talking with the person can aid in relaxation.

3. d. With guided imagery, the person creates a pleasant image in the mind, and focuses on that image and slowly becomes less aware of her pain.

4. c. Distraction works best with mild or moderate pain.

5. b. Between 25 and 50% of older adults living in the community have pain on a regular basis. The incidence is much higher (between 45-80%) for those living in nursing homes.

6. a. The person experiencing pain is the one who knows more about it than anyone else. Believe the person who reports pain.

7. c. Phantom pain is pain that is felt in a body part that is no longer present.

PAIN AND THE
OLDER PERSON

Everyone experiences pain at some point although pain is much more common among older persons. Between 25 and 50% of older adults living in the community have pain on a regular basis. The incidence is much higher (between 45-80%) for those living in nursing homes. One in five North Americans is affected by pain each day. Pain is the main reason for seeking health care services. Surveys in Canada indicate that over 18% of Canadians suffer from severe chronic pain and that chronic and severe pain sufferers are not always effectively treated.

WHAT IS PAIN?

Pain has been described as "an unpleasant sensory and emotional experience associated with actual or potential tissue damage." Pain is a very personal experience. You can't see or touch it. There are no tests to determine the presence or extent of pain. Pain is unique to each person. Two people in the same situation may experience pain in a different way. For example, one person may have mild pain from an injury, whereas another person may experience severe pain from the same type of injury. Pain can vary from one day to the next or from hour to hour. In nursing, pain is commonly considered to be whatever the person says it is.

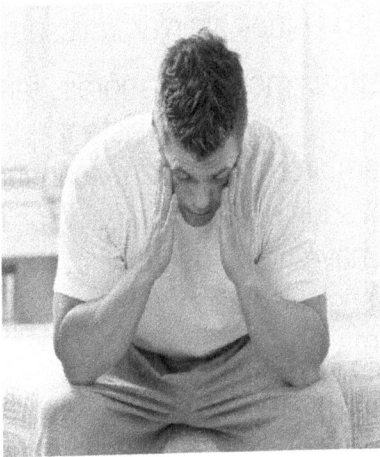

TYPES OF PAIN

This section discusses just some of the different ways to describe pain. Pain can be described as acute or chronic depending on how long it lasts. Acute pain is short-lived. It may result from surgery, a medical procedure, injury or disease. It responds well to treatment and fades as injured tissue heals.

Pain that lasts six months or more is termed chronic pain (sometimes called persistent pain). Chronic pain can stem from malignant (cancer related) or nonmalignant sources. Chronic pain can last for many years. It can have many negative outcomes such as depression, social isolation, decreased mobility, and sleep problems.

Two other terms you may hear are radiating pain and phantom pain. Radiating pain is pain that is felt in a site other than the source of the tissue damage. It spreads to other locations nearby. For example, pain from a gallbladder problem may be felt in the right side of the abdomen but the pain may spread to the back and the right shoulder. Phantom pain is pain that is felt in a body part that is no longer present. Phantom pain is commonly felt following the amputation of a limb.

CONSIDER FOR A MOMENT ...

Think about your own experiences with pain. Which of the four types of pain have you had?

MYTHS ABOUT PAIN

Pain can't be measured by any test or procedure. Perhaps because of this fact, many people with chronic pain are not believed. They may be labeled as complainers, drug addicts or attention seekers. A 1998 survey on pain found that 25% of chronic pain sufferers had trouble getting adequate medical help for their pain. One of the reasons given by the pain sufferers was that doctors had a poor understanding of pain management and did not take their pain seriously.

Sometimes friends, coworkers, family members and even healthcare workers hold false beliefs about pain. These false beliefs may lead people to be judgmental about the person with pain. People experiencing pain themselves may have false beliefs that affect their decisions about getting help. One study in Maryland found that 65% of respondents felt that pain was a natural part of aging and something they would just have to get used to. The table on the opposite page outlines some of the false beliefs or myths about pain that are common in society today.

Myths about pain

- Pain is a natural part of growing old
- Pain is uncomfortable but not harmful
- Only weak people admit to having pain
- Medication is only needed for severe pain
- Older people are not reliable reporters of their pain
- Chronic pain causes an increase in blood pressure and pulse
- Those who take narcotics for pain quickly become addicted to them
- Sleeping patients are not in pain
- People with dementia can't feel pain
- The use of narcotics will hasten death
- Older people have decreased sensation to pain

Many of these myths contribute to poor treatment and needless suffering for those with pain.

CONSIDER FOR A MOMENT ...
Do you know anyone who believes
in these myths? Do you believe in
any of them?

SIGNS AND SYMPTOMS OF PAIN

You need to get accurate information about the person's pain so that you can report it and so that he or she can receive proper treatment for the pain. The most reliable way to find out if someone is having pain is to ask him. The following are questions you should ask if someone is complaining of pain:

Where is the pain?

When did it start?

What does the pain feel like (describe the pain)?

How severe is the pain?

What do you believe may have caused the pain?

Pain can be described in a number of ways such as sharp, sore, aching, throbbing, discomfort, hurt, or a feeling of pressure or dullness. Health care workers have used different tools to help assess a person's pain. A numeric rating scale is one that is commonly used to check the severity of the pain. It asks the person to rate the pain from 0 (no pain) to 10 (worst pain).

Numeric Rating Scale

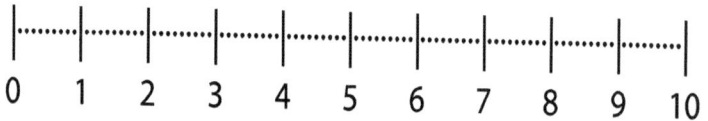

Numeric Rating Scale

```
|-------|-------|-------|-------|-------|-------|-------|-------|-------|-------|
0    1    2    3    4    5    6    7    8    9    10
```

Some older people find a numeric rating scale confusing. In those cases, they may be asked to describe the intensity of the pain in terms of "no pain", "mild pain", "moderate pain" or "severe pain."

Children are often presented with a series of pictures of faces. The faces (see the following page) show different expressions of pain level. The child is asked to point to the picture that best describes the pain intensity. The child is asked to choose the face that best describes their own pain and record the appropriate number. The rating scale is recommended for children 3 years and older. It can be used with older adults.

Wong-Baker FACES Pain Rating Scale

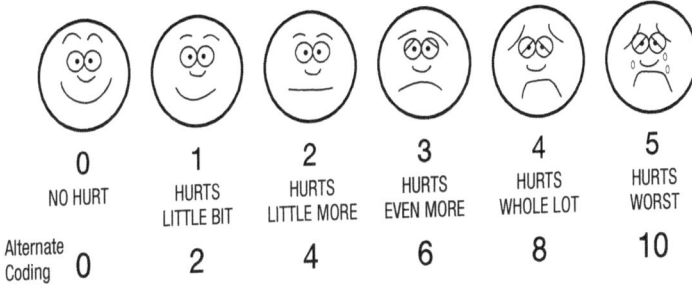

0	1	2	3	4	5
NO HURT	HURTS LITTLE BIT	HURTS LITTLE MORE	HURTS EVEN MORE	HURTS WHOLE LOT	HURTS WORST

Alternate Coding 0 2 4 6 8 10

The body responds to pain in certain common ways such as pale skin, perspiring, nausea, vomiting, increase in pulse, respirations, and blood pressure. Not everyone shows all of these symptoms. For example, pulse, respirations, and blood pressure may be normal if the pain has been present for some time. These vital signs may not increase if the person with pain is elderly.

BEHAVIORS THAT MAY INDICATE PAIN

Certain behaviors are common when people have pain. Remember, these are common responses to pain. They are not always present:

- Grimacing
- Being still
- Holding or rubbing a body part
- Restlessness, agitation, irritability
- Changes in speech (e.g. unusually loud or quiet)
- Groaning, moaning, grunting, gasping, crying, screaming

Persons with chronic pain may be tired and sleep more than usual. They may not eat well and become depressed. Sometimes the first signs you may notice are related to functional status. There may be changes in their ability to walk, feed, wash, dress, and use the bathroom. A person who used to love attending social events may now spend more time alone. Movements may become slow and rigid. Sudden onset of confusion is a common sign of infection among older people. It can also be a sign of poorly controlled pain.

Sometimes your loved ones will tell you they are having pain. At other times, they may not be willing or able to tell you about their pain. Observation is even more important in those cases. Observe the person for possible signs of pain such as the ones noted above. Observe for other unusual signs and symptoms. If your loved one is living in a health care facility, pulse and blood pressure should be monitored and pain observations should be documented.

FACTORS AFFECTING PAIN

Pain is complex and people react to it in different ways. A number of factors affect how people experience and react to pain.

Age

Developmental stage affects the way that people react to pain. Young children do not understand pain, may not know the words to be able to describe it and have trouble 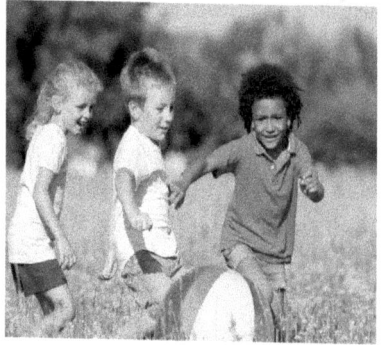 coping with it. Older people have had experience with pain but may have false beliefs that affect their attitude towards it. As well, older people are more likely to have chronic diseases that cause pain. Pain can stem from more than one chronic condition at a time, making it hard to identify the source of pain and to treat it effectively.

Culture

Don't assume that the person who does not cry or moan is not in severe pain. In many cultures it is acceptable for persons with pain to become very vocal. In others, however, silence is the norm. Culture has a strong impact on how people respond to pain. It is important to ask the person how he or she usually reacts when in pain.

Past experience with pain

Past experience with pain can impact how a person reacts to the current episode. If previous bouts of pain were severe and hard to control, the person may react to the onset of a new incident with anxiety and fear. If, on the other hand, past episodes were mild and easily controlled, she may be fairly relaxed about this episode. People who have never had much experience with pain are often fearful. They don't know what to expect and fear that they won't be able to cope.

Attention

The extent to which a person thinks about pain affects how severe it seems. Even mild pain can seem worse if the person focuses on it. People in pain who are awake at night with little to distract them often find the pain more severe.

Meaning of pain

Pain may seem worse depending on the meaning attached to it. Some people see pain as a punishment for past deeds. For others, pain may be a sign of a serious illness or the spread of an existing disease.

Anxiety

Pain causes a person to be anxious. On the other hand, anxiety makes pain seem worse. It can be more difficult to control pain in a highly anxious person.

Rest

Fatigue and lack of sleep have a negative impact on pain control. Pain always seems more manageable when a person is well rested. More people feel pain at the end of the day when they are tired rather than in the morning.

Coping style

Over time, some people are able to find ways to cope with their pain. Coping methods may include relaxing, talking to family members, or distraction. Others have poor coping resources for pain.

Support from family and friends

Close contact with friends and loved ones can go a long way to helping the client with pain. People without social support are more lonely and afraid and have more pain.

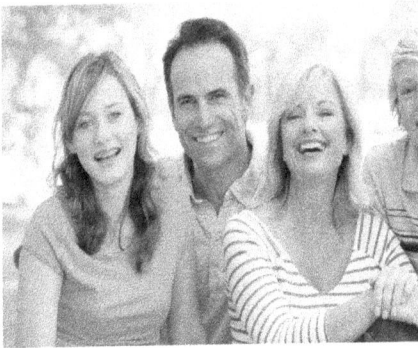

Gender

Gender differences arise from society influences, hormones and genes. Society in general expects males to show a 'stiff upper lip' when in pain. Research has shown that women are more sensitive to pain just before menstruation. As well, a pain gene may influence the extent that pain is perceived.

THE OLDER ADULT

Pain is not a normal part of aging although it is more common among older persons. It is generally believed that the ability to perceive pain does not decrease with age.

Older people are prone to accidents such as falls that result in fractures or sprains that cause acute pain. Chronic pain is very common and may stem from a number of conditions. Chronic pain from nonmalignant sources often stems from arthritis, back pain or a condition called fibromyalgia. Fibromyalgia causes aching, stiffness and fatigue in muscles and soft tissues. It also creates problems with sleep. The most common reason for chronic pain in older adults is osteoarthritis.

Death and disease narrow down the list of social contacts for older people. Pain makes it difficult for them to spend time with the few remaining people who are close to them. The resulting boredom and lack of social contact leads to depression and decreased ability to cope with the pain.

Pain may cause the older person to be less mobile which leads to problems with bathing, dressing and walking. Over time, the person may become more dependent on others for all aspects of daily living.

Sometimes it's hard to find the source of the pain. Older persons may have more than one chronic condition that causes pain. They may think that pain is related to the first condition and not seek help with the second problem. Multiple chronic conditions make pain management more complex.

Sometimes people experiencing pain do not seek help for it. They may feel that it is normal so not worth reporting or they may not have the money to pay for health care products and services such as pills, treatments, equipment, and so on.

PAIN AND THE PERSON WITH DEMENTIA

As noted earlier, pain is considered to be whatever the person says it is. Many older people, however, have conditions (e.g. stroke, Parkinson's disease, dementia) that make it difficult for them to report pain or to let others know if pain treatments have worked.

Dementia describes a group of symptoms caused by a variety of disorders. The disorders cause a decline in mental and cognitive function over time.

Alzheimer's disease (AD) is the most common form of dementia. AD affects thought, memory and language. After the age of 65, the incidence of AD doubles every 5 years. It has been estimated that over

4.5 million Americans have AD. There are currently about half a million Canadians living with Alzheimer's disease or a related dementia. Estimates for Canada are that one in 11 persons in the 65+ age category has the disease. As well, the incidence in persons 85 years and more is 25%.

Very little is known about pain in people with dementia. As the condition worsens, those affected by dementia may not be able to report pain. They may not even be able to recognize the presence of pain. People with dementia are less likely to be treated for pain than those with no mental impairment. Just because they cannot report pain, however, does not mean it is not present. More research needs to be done in this area.

People with a minor or moderate degree of mental impairment should be asked questions about their pain. As the mental impairment worsens, you will have to rely upon what you observe (signs and symptoms) to find out if a person is in pain. You must be very observant in order to detect cues that may show the person is in pain. Aggression may be a sign of pain in people with dementia.

PAIN MANAGEMENT

False beliefs lead to poor management of pain. Many caregivers believe that pain among older people is 'normal', something that is a natural part of aging and that cannot be controlled. Pain is a sign of injury or disease. It is never a normal process. The American Pain Foundation has outlined a number of rights called the "Pain Care Bill of Rights" (see the following page) that people with pain should insist upon receiving. The Chronic Pain Association of Canada outlines similar rights on their website

http://www.chronicpaincanada.com

PAIN CARE BILL OF RIGHTS

As a person with pain, you have
the right to:

- Be believed when you say you have pain

- Be treated with dignity and compassion
  by healthcare workers

- Have your pain assessed and effectively
  treated

- Be fully informed about your pain, including
  possible side effects of treatments

- Actively participate in decisions about
  managing your pain

- Have your pain reassessed regularly

- Seek changes in treatment if pain persists

- See a pain specialist if your pain continues

- Have your questions answered

The primary goal of pain management should be to prevent, rather than lessen, pain. Pain management should be specific for the person. What works for one individual may not work for another. Follow treatment advice and the person's care plan to promote comfort and manage pain. A combination of drugs and other methods works best to manage pain. You may not be involved in assisting with all of the methods discussed in this section although you may find it helpful to know about them.

Medications

Medications may be ordered regularly over a 24-hour period for pain that persists. Pain medication is often prescribed in a lower dose for older persons due to a change in drug absorption time with age. Some of the medications used for pain medication in young or middle-aged adults are not recommended for use in older adults.

Complementary/alternative therapies

Various complementary and alternative therapies have been used with success to help the person with pain. Complementary therapies are ones that are used in addition to traditional medical treatments. Alternative therapies are used in place of a medical treatment. Some of these methods are touch, acupuncture and acupressure, biofeedback, meditation, guided imagery and self-hypnosis.

Touch

Back rubs have been used by nurses to promote rest and comfort since Florence Nightingale's day. Therapeutic touch is another technique involving the hands. This method includes placing the hands on or near the body with the intent to heal. Therapeutic touch works well in some but not all cases.

Acupuncture and acupressure

Acupuncture is an ancient technique that began in Asia. It involves using long fine needles at certain points in the body to open energy pathways. Acupressure involves applying pressure to these energy points to relieve pain. Both methods have been used with success to control chronic pain.

Biofeedback

Biofeedback is a training technique that lets a person gain control over some body functions.

Meditation

Meditation is a technique in which the person focuses his thoughts on a word or phrase blocking out all other thoughts. Meditation has been shown to lower blood pressure and reduce stress.

Guided imagery

With guided imagery, the person creates a pleasant image in the mind, and focuses on that image until he slowly becomes less aware of pain. It uses the power of the mind to reduce stress and anxiety.

Self-hypnosis

Self-hypnosis involves intense concentration on a relaxing image. The person becomes conditioned to relax whenever she thinks about the image.

Cutaneous nerve stimulation

This method involves stimulation of the skin to lessen pain. It can involve massage, vibration, heat, cold or ointments. Heat and cold are used to short circuit the flow of pain impulses to the pain center of the brain. Heat and cold treatments should be used with great care in older persons. Their skin is very sensitive and feeling in their extremities may be reduced.

Transcutaneous electrical nerve stimulation

This method involves the placement of electrodes over the pain site. These electrodes release an electrical current and prevent pain signals from reaching the brain's pain center.

Distraction

Distraction works best with mild or moderate pain. Examples of methods used to distract are humor, music, conversation and television. Distraction works by getting the person to focus on something other than his pain.

Relaxation

Relaxation quiets the mind and body, relieving anxiety and stress. Guided imagery and meditation help produce a relaxed state. So does deep, slow breathing done while relaxing various muscle groups.

Communication

Encourage your loved one to share her thoughts, fears and feelings about pain. Wait 30 minutes after pain medication before starting any treatments that may cause pain. The wait period gives the medication time to work. Be supportive. Remember, the person experiencing pain is the expert in his or her own pain, and should be believed.

Rest and sleep

Rest and sleep are very important for people who are not feeling well. They should avoid caffeine in late afternoon and early evening. Establish a night time routine. Help create calm and relaxed surroundings. Ensure the area is quiet. Other measures to use to promote comfort and rest include:

- Play soft music
- Darken the room
- Give a back massage
- Use proper positioning
- Use blankets for warmth
- Be flexible about bedtime
- Handle the person with care
- Sit and talk with him to aid in relaxation
- Advise the person to avoid physical activity before bedtime
- Provide assistance with toileting as needed and particularly before naps and bedtime

CONSIDER FOR A MOMENT ...

Can you think of any other measures that can be used to promote comfort, rest and sleep?

CASE EXAMPLE

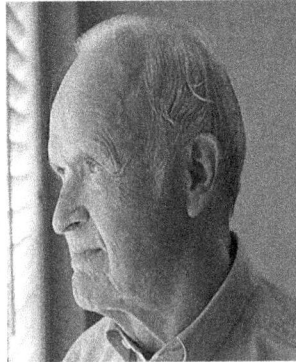

Mr. Andrews is 75 years old and lives at home. He has had pain from osteoarthritis for over 20 years. He has been prescribed medication for pain but reports that he doesn't always take it as he doesn't want to 'get addicted' to drugs. Mr. Andrews has one son who lives far away and seldom visits. Most of his other relatives and friends have passed away so he spends a lot of time alone.

He used to enjoy walking, painting and gardening but can no longer do those things due to the worsening of his joints. He has no other hobbies or interests. He seldom complains. When questioned, however, he tells you that his pain is worse at night. He sleeps poorly and is tired all the time.

What type of pain does Mr. Andrews have?

Which of the factors discussed in the section "Factors affecting pain" are present in this scenario?

YOUR ANSWERS TO CASE EXAMPLE

SUGGESTED ANSWERS TO CASE EXAMPLE

What type of pain does Mr. Andrews have?

Mr. Andrews has had pain from osteoarthritis for over 20 years. Pain that lasts six months or more is called chronic pain.

Which of the factors discussed in the section "Factors affecting pain" are present in this scenario?

The factors affecting pain that are present in this scenario are:

Age

Older people are more likely to have chronic diseases such as osteoarthritis that cause pain. As well, although older people have had experience with pain, they often have false beliefs that affect their attitude towards it. Mr. Andrews doesn't always take his medication as he is afraid of becoming addicted to it.

Attention

Mr. Andrews finds the pain worse at night. People who are awake at night with little to distract them often find the pain more severe.

Rest

Fatigue and lack of sleep make pain seem worse.

Support from family and friends

People without social support are more lonely and afraid and have more pain.

Gender

Society in general expects that males will not express their pain. Mr. Andrews seldom complains about pain.

CONCLUSION

Pain is a common problem for older adults and has the potential to cause many negative outcomes such as depression, social isolation, decreased mobility and sleep problems.

Myths about pain persist even among caregivers. These myths contribute to poor treatment and needless suffering for those with pain. The most reliable way to find out if someone is having pain is to ask the person.

Certain behaviors are common when people have pain and caregivers need to watch for signs that may indicate pain. A number of factors impact the way that people experience and react to pain. Some people are unable to talk about their pain so that observation becomes even more important.

A combination of drugs and other measures works best to control pain although pain management is individual to the person. Rest and sleep are very important aspects of pain management.

SOME HELPFUL RESOURCES

Below are web sites from various pain-related organizations. These web sites provide important information to persons affected by pain and/or to caregivers.

American Academy of Hospice and Palliative Medicine (AAHPM) http://www.aahpm.org

American Academy of Pain Managementhttp://www.aapainmanage.org

American Chronic Pain Association (ACPA) http://www.theacpa.org

American Pain Foundation (APF) http://www.painfoundation.org

American Pain Society (APS) http://www.ampainsoc.org

American Society for Pain Management Nursing (ASPMN) http://www.aspmn.org

Chronic Pain Association of Canada (CPAC) http://www.chronicpaincanada.com

International Association for the Study of Pain (IASP) http://www.iasp-pain.org

National Center for Complementary and Alternative Medicine (NCCAM) http://nccam.nih.gov

National Pain Education Council (NPEC) http://www.npecweb.org

Nurse Healers-Professional Associates International (NHPAI) http://www.therapeutic-touch.org

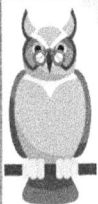

CHECK YOUR KNOWLEDGE

1. Define acute, chronic, radiating and phantom pain.

2. List four common myths about pain.

3. What behaviors are commonly observed in persons with pain?

4. Identify three factors that affect how people react to pain.

5. Discuss two nondrug methods that can be used to manage pain.

6. Describe four strategies that you can use to promote rest and sleep in people with pain.

TEST YOURSELF

Please circle to indicate the best answer:

1. The person you are caring for is clutching her abdomen and complaining of pain. Her pulse, respirations and blood pressure are normal. It is most likely that:

a. She is elderly

b. She is confused

c. Her pain is phantom pain

d. She is imagining the pain

2. Which statement about pain is a myth?

a. Pain cannot be objectively measured

b. Medication is only needed for severe pain

c. The person with chronic pain may sleep more than usual

d. Sudden confusion can be a sign of poorly controlled pain in older adults

3. Which factor makes pain management among older adults more difficult?

a. They have decreased sensation to pain

b. They may have multiple chronic conditions

c. They quickly become addicted to medications

d. They are not reliable reporters of their pain

4. Which statement about pain and dementia is true?

a. People with dementia have diminished pain sensation

b. People with dementia may strike out at others when in pain

c. Through research we now know a great deal about pain in people with dementia

d. People with dementia are just as likely to be treated for pain as those with no mental impairment

5. What is the most common reason for chronic pain in older adults?

a. Headaches

b. Back pain

c. Fibromyalgia

d. Osteoarthritis

6. You must do mouth care in the morning on someone who finds the treatment painful. You should:

a. Skip mouth care for the day

b. Begin the treatment 30 minutes before pain medication is due

c. Begin the treatment as soon as the pain medication has been given

d. Wait 30 minutes after pain medication has been given to let the medicine work

7. Which measure is a good example of distraction?

a. Humor

b. Keeping the lights on at night

c. Following a regular routine for care

d. Keeping the room at a comfortable temperature

ANSWERS:

1. **a.** Pulse, respirations, and blood pressure may be normal if the pain has been present for some time. These vital signs may not increase if the person with pain is elderly.

2. **b.** It is a widely-held myth that medication is only needed for severe pain.

3. **b.** Older people are more likely to have chronic diseases that cause pain. Pain can stem from more than one chronic condition at a time, making it hard to identify the source of pain and to treat it effectively.

4. **b.** Aggression may be a sign of pain in people with dementia.

5. **d.** The most common reason for chronic pain in older adults is osteoarthritis.

6. **d.** Wait 30 minutes after pain medication before starting any treatments that may cause pain.

7. **a.** Humor is an example of a method used to distract someone from his pain. Others are music, conversation and television.

REFERENCES

Alzheimer's Association (2006). Causes. Retrieved May 17, 2006, from http://www.alz.org/AboutAD/causes.asp

American Pain Foundation (March, 2005). Pain facts. Retrieved June 11, 2006, http://www.painfoundation.org/page.asp?file=Library/PainSurveys.htm

American Pain Foundation (2003). Pain Care Bill of Rights. Retrieved June 12, 2006, http://www.painfoundation.org/page.asp?file=Publications/Index.htm

Chronic Pain Association of Canada (2006). Pain facts. Retrieved June 11, 2006, http://www.chronicpaincanada.com/

Ebersole, P., Hess, P., Touhy, T., & Jett, K. (2005). Gerontological nursing & healthy aging (2nd ed.). St. Louis: Mosby.

Ebersole, P., Hess, P., & Luggen, A. (2004). Toward healthy aging (6th ed.). St. Louis: Mosby.

Hockenberry, M. J., Wilson, D., & Winkelstein, M.L. (2005, p.1259). Wong's essentials of pediatric nursing, ed. 7. St. Louis: Mosby.

Horgas, A. & Elliott, A. (2004). Pain assessment and management in persons with dementia. Nursing Clinics of North America, 39 (3), 593-606.

International Association for the Study of Pain (IASP). (November 9, 2004). Pain Terms. Retrieved June 9, 2006, http://www.iasp-pain.org/terms-p.html#Pain

Jarvis, C. (2004). Physical examination and health assessment (4th ed.). St. Louis: Saunders.

Potter, P., & Perry, A. (2001). Canadian fundamentals of nursing (2nd ed.). Ross-Kerr, J., & Wood, M. J. (Canadian editors). St. Louis: Mosby.

Renn, C. & Dorsey, S. (2005). The physiology and processing of pain: A review. American Association of Critical Care Nurses, 16 (3), 277-290.

Siciliano, P. & Burrage, R. (2005). Chronic pain in the elderly: A continuing education program for certified nursing assistants. Geriatric Nursing, 26 (4), 252-258.

Snyder, M. & Lindquist, R. (May 31, 2001). Issues in complementary therapies: How we got to where we are. Online Journal of Issues in Nursing, 6 (2), Manuscript 1. Retrieved June 16, 2006 http://www.nursingworld.org/ojin/topic15/tpc15_1.htm

Sorrentino, S. (2004). Mosby's Canadian textbook for the support worker. Toronto, ON: Mosby.

www.ingramcontent.com/pod-product-compliance
Lightning Source LLC
Chambersburg PA
CBHW071348200326
41520CB00013B/3154